TYPE 1 DIABETES COOKBOOK FOR ADULTS

Delicious Recipes & Meal Plans for Balanced Blood Sugar Management

T. John

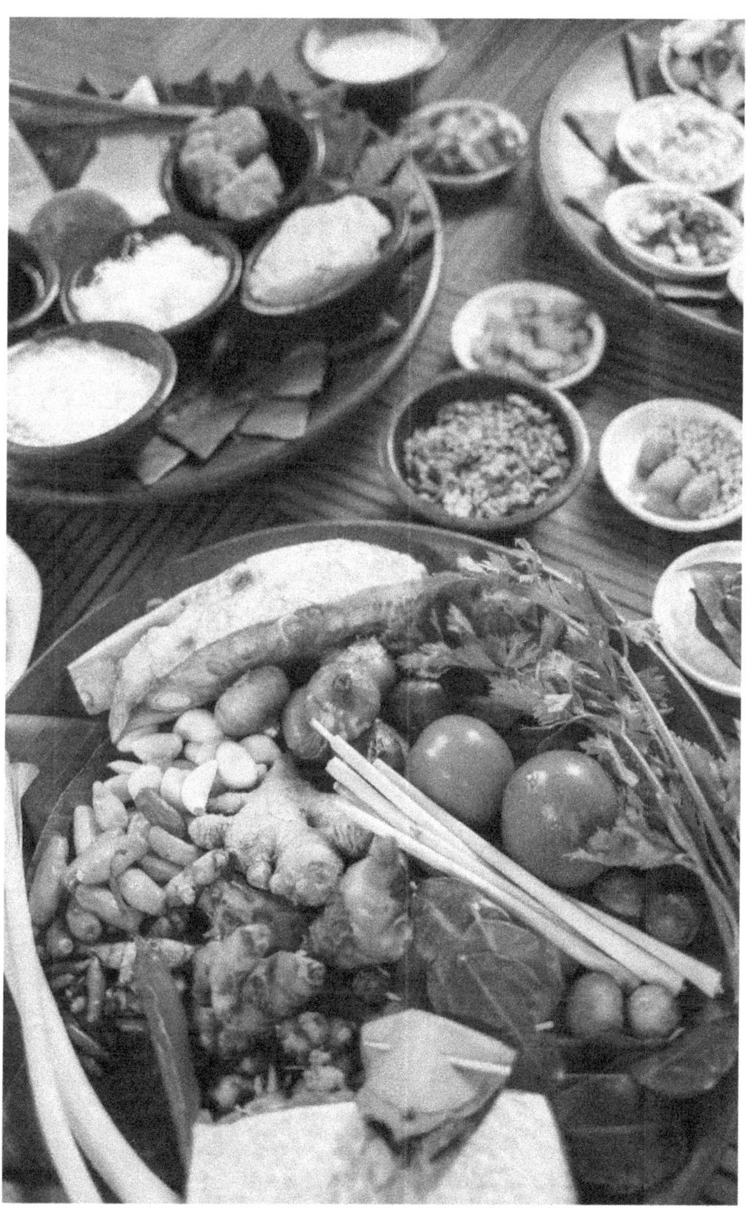

TABLE OF CONTENTS

Chapter 3: Lunch Recipes 46

Chapter 6: Desserts 109

INTRODUCTION

Type 1 diabetes (T1D) can feel like a whirlwind at times. Your body doesn't produce insulin, a hormone crucial for regulating blood sugar. This means managing your diet becomes an essential part of your daily routine. But fear not, with a little planning and knowledge, you can create a delicious and healthy lifestyle that keeps your blood sugar in check.

Understanding Type 1 Diabetes: The Body's Balancing Act

Imagine your body is a giant kitchen. Food is the fuel, and insulin is the chef. The chef breaks down the food into sugar (glucose), the body's primary energy source. In T1D, your kitchen lacks a chef, so the sugar builds up instead of being used efficiently. This can lead to a myriad of health problems if left unchecked.

Diet: Your Secret Weapon for Blood Sugar Control

The good news is you can influence how much sugar enters your bloodstream through your diet. Different foods affect blood sugar levels at varying rates. Here's where your inner food scientist comes in!

- **Carb Counting**: Carbohydrates are the biggest influencers of blood sugar. Learn to estimate carbs in your meals – a skill that becomes second nature over time. This helps you match your insulin dose to the incoming sugar.
- **Fiber is Your Friend**: Opt for complex carbs like whole grains and vegetables. These are packed with fiber, which slows down sugar absorption, preventing spikes.
- **Protein Power:** Include protein sources like lean meats, fish, and legumes in every meal. Protein helps you feel fuller for longer and provides a steady energy release.

- **Healthy Fats:** Don't fear fats! Healthy fats like avocado and nuts keep you satiated and add flavor. Just be mindful of portion sizes.

Meal Planning: The Roadmap to Success

Planning your meals ahead of time is a game-changer. Here are some tips to get you started:

- **Involve the Whole Crew:** Get your family or friends on board. Explore healthy recipes together and make meal prep a fun activity.
- **Variety is Key:** Don't get stuck in a rut! Explore different cuisines and experiment with new ingredients. There's a whole world of delicious healthy food waiting to be discovered.
- **Portion Control is Essential:** Use measuring cups and spoons to ensure you're not overdoing it. Consider using a visual guide like the plate method to create balanced meals.

- **Don't Forget Snacks**: Plan healthy snacks throughout the day to keep your blood sugar levels stable and avoid unhealthy cravings.

Blood Sugar Management: The Art of Monitoring

Monitoring your blood sugar regularly is vital. It gives you valuable insights into how your body reacts to different foods and activities.

- **Befriend Your Blood Glucose Meter**: Become comfortable with checking your blood sugar before meals, after meals, and at other times throughout the day as advised by your doctor.
- **Track and Analyze**: Keep a log of your blood sugar readings, meals, and insulin doses. This allows you and your doctor to identify patterns and adjust your approach as needed.

Remember: You are not alone on this journey. With a little planning and the right knowledge, you can conquer type 1 diabetes and live a full, vibrant life.

Chapter 1: 30 Day Meal Plan

Week 1:

Day 1:

- Breakfast: Avocado and Egg Breakfast Bowl
- Lunch: Grilled Chicken Caesar Salad
- Dinner: Baked Salmon with Asparagus
- Snack: Veggie Sticks with Hummus
- Dessert: Berry and Yogurt Popsicles

Day 2:

- Breakfast: Greek Yogurt Parfait with Berries
- Lunch: Turkey and Hummus Wrap
- Dinner: Spaghetti Squash with Turkey Bolognese
- Snack: Apple Slices with Almond Butter
- Dessert: Dark Chocolate Covered Strawberries

Day 3:

- Breakfast: Spinach and Feta Omelette
- Lunch: Quinoa and Black Bean Salad

- Dinner: Lemon Garlic Chicken with Roasted Vegetables
- Snack: Cheese and Whole Grain Crackers
- Dessert: Sugar-Free Cheesecake Bites

Day 4:

- Breakfast: Overnight Oats with Chia Seeds
- Lunch: Asian Chicken Lettuce Wraps
- Dinner: Cauliflower Fried Rice with Shrimp
- Snack: Hard-Boiled Eggs with Mustard
- Dessert: Almond Flour Chocolate Chip Cookies

Day 5:

- Breakfast: Whole Wheat Pancakes with Sugar-Free Syrup
- Lunch: Mediterranean Chickpea Salad
- Dinner: Stuffed Bell Peppers with Ground Turkey
- Snack: Mixed Nuts and Seeds
- Dessert: Greek Yogurt with Honey and Almonds

Day 6:

- Breakfast: Veggie Breakfast Burrito

- Lunch: Veggie Stir-Fry with Tofu

- Dinner: Beef and Broccoli Stir-Fry

- Snack: Edamame with Sea Salt

- Dessert: Chia Seed Pudding with Berries

Day 7:

- Breakfast: Quinoa Breakfast Porridge

- Lunch: Tuna Salad Stuffed Avocado

- Dinner: Veggie and Bean Chili

- Snack: Cucumber Slices with Cream Cheese

- Dessert: Baked Apple Slices with Cinnamon

Week 2:

Day 8:

- Breakfast: Almond Butter Toast with Banana Slices

- Lunch: Caprese Panini with Whole Grain Bread

- Dinner: Grilled Swordfish with Mango Salsa

- Snack: Baked Kale Chips

- Dessert: Banana Nice Cream with Peanut Butter

Day 9:

- Breakfast: Breakfast Muffin Tin Frittatas

- Lunch: Lentil and Vegetable Soup

- Dinner: Zucchini Noodles with Pesto and Grilled Chicken

- Snack: Cottage Cheese with Pineapple Chunks

- Dessert: Coconut Flour Blueberry Muffins

Day 10:

- Breakfast: Smoked Salmon and Cream Cheese Bagel

- Lunch: Shrimp and Quinoa Salad

- Dinner: Pork Tenderloin with Roasted Brussels Sprouts

- Snack: Mini Caprese Skewers

- Dessert: Avocado Chocolate Mousse

Day 11:

- Breakfast: Cottage Cheese Pancakes

- Lunch: Chicken and Veggie Kebabs

- Dinner: Turkey Meatballs with Marinara Sauce

- Snack: Roasted Chickpeas

- Dessert: Lemon Poppy Seed Cake Bites

Day 12:

- Breakfast: Tofu Scramble with Veggies
- Lunch: Egg Salad Lettuce Wraps
- Dinner: Ratatouille with Quinoa
- Snack: Turkey and Cheese Roll-Ups
- Dessert: Pistachio Cranberry Energy Bites

Day 13:

- Breakfast: Breakfast Quinoa Bowl with Nuts and Fruit
- Lunch: Turkey and Vegetable Skewers
- Dinner: Chicken Curry with Cauliflower Rice
- Snack: Avocado Salsa with Baked Tortilla Chips
- Dessert: Pumpkin Pie Chia Pudding

Day 14:

- Breakfast: Baked Egg Cups with Spinach and Tomatoes
- Lunch: Greek Salad with Grilled Halloumi
- Dinner: Beef Stir-Fry with Ginger and Snap Peas
- Snack: Stuffed Mushrooms with Spinach and Feta
- Dessert: Carrot Cake Oatmeal Cookies

Week 3:

Day 15:

- Breakfast: Zucchini and Bacon Breakfast Hash
- Lunch: Cauliflower Crust Pizza with Salad
- Dinner: Baked Cod with Herbed Quinoa
- Snack: Veggie Sticks with Hummus
- Dessert: Chocolate Avocado Pudding

Day 16:

- Breakfast: Avocado and Egg Breakfast Bowl
- Lunch: Grilled Chicken Caesar Salad
- Dinner: Spaghetti Squash with Turkey Bolognese
- Snack: Greek Yogurt Dip with Fresh Veggies
- Dessert: Berry and Yogurt Popsicles

Day 17:

- Breakfast: Greek Yogurt Parfait with Berries
- Lunch: Turkey and Hummus Wrap
- Dinner: Lemon Garlic Chicken with Roasted Vegetables
- Snack: Apple Slices with Almond Butter
- Dessert: Dark Chocolate Covered Strawberries

Day 18:

- Breakfast: Spinach and Feta Omelette
- Lunch: Quinoa and Black Bean Salad
- Dinner: Cauliflower Fried Rice with Shrimp
- Snack: Cheese and Whole Grain Crackers
- Dessert: Sugar-Free Cheesecake Bites

Day 19:

- Breakfast: Overnight Oats with Chia Seeds
- Lunch: Asian Chicken Lettuce Wraps
- Dinner: Stuffed Bell Peppers with Ground Turkey
- Snack: Hard-Boiled Eggs with Mustard
- Dessert: Almond Flour Chocolate Chip Cookies

Day 20:

- Breakfast: Whole Wheat Pancakes with Sugar-Free Syrup
- Lunch: Mediterranean Chickpea Salad
- Dinner: Beef and Broccoli Stir-Fry
- Snack: Mixed Nuts and Seeds
- Dessert: Greek Yogurt with Honey and Almonds

Day 21:

- Breakfast: Veggie Breakfast Burrito
- Lunch: Veggie Stir-Fry with Tofu
- Dinner: Grilled Swordfish with Mango Salsa
- Snack: Edamame with Sea Salt
- Dessert: Chia Seed Pudding with Berries

Week 4:

Day 22:

- Breakfast: Quinoa Breakfast Porridge
- Lunch: Tuna Salad Stuffed Avocado
- Dinner: Veggie and Bean Chili
- Snack: Cucumber Slices with Cream Cheese
- Dessert: Baked Apple Slices with Cinnamon

Day 23:

- Breakfast: Almond Butter Toast with Banana Slices
- Lunch: Caprese Panini with Whole Grain Bread
- Dinner: Pork Tenderloin with Roasted Brussels Sprouts
- Snack: Baked Kale Chips
- Dessert: Banana Nice Cream with Peanut Butter

Day 24:

- Breakfast: Breakfast Muffin Tin Frittatas
- Lunch: Lentil and Vegetable Soup
- Dinner: Zucchini Noodles with Pesto and Grilled Chicken
- Snack: Cottage Cheese with Pineapple Chunks
- Dessert: Coconut Flour Blueberry Muffins

Day 25:

- Breakfast: Smoked Salmon and Cream Cheese Bagel
- Lunch: Shrimp and Quinoa Salad
- Dinner: Turkey Meatballs with Marinara Sauce
- Snack: Mini Caprese Skewers
- Dessert: Avocado Chocolate Mousse

Day 26:

- Breakfast: Cottage Cheese Pancakes
- Lunch: Chicken and Veggie Kebabs
- Dinner: Ratatouille with Quinoa
- Snack: Roasted Chickpeas
- Dessert: Lemon Poppy Seed Cake Bites

Day 27:

- Breakfast: Tofu Scramble with Veggies
- Lunch: Egg Salad Lettuce Wraps
- Dinner: Chicken Curry with Cauliflower Rice
- Snack: Avocado Salsa with Baked Tortilla Chips
- Dessert: Pumpkin Pie Chia Pudding

Day 28:

- Breakfast: Breakfast Quinoa Bowl with Nuts and Fruit
- Lunch: Turkey and Vegetable Skewers
- Dinner: Beef Stir-Fry with Ginger and Snap Peas
- Snack: Stuffed Mushrooms with Spinach and Feta
- Dessert: Carrot Cake Oatmeal Cookies

Day 29:

- Breakfast: Baked Egg Cups with Spinach and Tomatoes
- Lunch: Greek Salad with Grilled Halloumi
- Dinner: Cauliflower Crust Pizza with Salad
- Snack: Veggie Sticks with Hummus
- Dessert: Chocolate Avocado Pudding

Day 30:

- Breakfast: Zucchini and Bacon Breakfast Hash
- Lunch: Cauliflower Crust Pizza with Salad
- Dinner: Baked Cod with Herbed Quinoa
- Snack: Greek Yogurt Dip with Fresh Veggies
- Dessert: Pistachio Cranberry Energy Bites

Chapter 2: Breakfast Recipes

These breakfast recipes are designed to fuel your body and keep your blood sugar stable throughout the day. From savory omelettes to satisfying oatmeal bowls, there's something here for everyone. Each recipe is packed with wholesome ingredients and easy to prepare, making it perfect for busy mornings.

Avocado and Egg Breakfast Bowl

Ingredients:

- 1 ripe avocado
- 2 eggs
- Salt and pepper to taste
- Optional toppings: cherry tomatoes, feta cheese, cilantro

Instructions:

1. Cut the avocado in half and remove the pit.
2. Scoop out a bit of the flesh to make room for the eggs.

3. Crack an egg into each avocado half.

4. Season with salt and pepper.

5. Bake in the oven at 375°F (190°C) for 15-20 minutes, or until the eggs are set.

6. Top with your favorite toppings and enjoy!

Nutrition Information:

- Calories: 320
- Protein: 14g
- Carbohydrates: 14g
- Fat: 24g
- Fiber: 10g
- Sugar: 1g
- Portion size: 1 serving

Greek Yogurt Parfait with Berries

Ingredients:

- 1 cup Greek yogurt
- 1/2 cup mixed berries (such as strawberries, blueberries, raspberries)
- 1/4 cup granola
- Honey (optional)

Instructions:

1. In a glass or bowl, layer Greek yogurt, berries, and granola.
2. Repeat layers until ingredients are used up.
3. Drizzle with honey if desired.
4. Serve immediately and enjoy!

Nutrition Information:

- Calories: 250
- Protein: 18g
- Carbohydrates: 30g
- Fat: 7g
- Fiber: 5g
- Sugar: 15g
- Portion size: 1 serving

Spinach and Feta Omelette

Ingredients:

- 2 eggs
- Handful of fresh spinach
- 1/4 cup crumbled feta cheese
- Salt and pepper to taste

Instructions:

1. Beat the eggs in a bowl and season with salt and pepper.
2. Heat a non-stick skillet over medium heat and add the beaten eggs.
3. Cook for 2-3 minutes, then add the spinach and feta cheese on one half of the omelette.
4. Fold the other half of the omelette over the filling and cook for another 2-3 minutes, or until the eggs are set.
5. Slide onto a plate and serve hot.

Nutrition Information:

- Calories: 280
- Protein: 20g
- Carbohydrates: 4g
- Fat: 20g
- Fiber: 2g
- Sugar: 1g
- Portion size: 1 serving

Overnight Oats with Chia Seeds

Ingredients:

- 1/2 cup rolled oats
- 1 tablespoon chia seeds
- 1/2 cup almond milk
- 1/4 teaspoon vanilla extract
- 1 tablespoon honey (optional)
- Fresh fruit for topping (such as sliced strawberries, banana, or blueberries)

Instructions:

1. In a jar or bowl, combine rolled oats, chia seeds, almond milk, vanilla extract, and honey (if using).
2. Stir well to combine.
3. Cover and refrigerate overnight, or for at least 4 hours.
4. In the morning, give the oats a stir and top with your favorite fresh fruit.
5. Enjoy cold or heat in the microwave for a warm breakfast option.

Nutrition Information:

- Calories: 280
- Protein: 8g
- Carbohydrates: 40g
- Fat: 10g
- Fiber: 10g
- Sugar: 10g
- Portion size: 1 serving

Whole Wheat Pancakes with Sugar-Free Syrup

Ingredients:

- 1 cup whole wheat flour
- 1 tablespoon baking powder
- 1 tablespoon sugar substitute
- 1 egg
- 1 cup almond milk
- 1 tablespoon vegetable oil
- Sugar-free syrup for serving

Instructions:

1. In a bowl, whisk together whole wheat flour, baking powder, and sugar substitute.
2. In a separate bowl, beat the egg and then stir in almond milk and vegetable oil.
3. Pour the wet ingredients into the dry ingredients and stir until just combined. Be careful not to overmix.
4. Heat a non-stick skillet over medium heat and lightly grease with oil or cooking spray.
5. Pour 1/4 cup of batter onto the skillet for each pancake.
6. Cook until bubbles form on the surface, then flip and cook for another 1-2 minutes.
7. Serve hot with sugar-free syrup.

Nutrition Information:

- Calories: 220
- Protein: 8g
- Carbohydrates: 30g
- Fat: 8g
- Fiber: 6g
- Sugar: 1g

- Portion size: 2 pancakes with syrup

Veggie Breakfast Burrito

Ingredients:

- 2 large whole wheat tortillas
- 4 eggs, scrambled
- 1/2 cup black beans, drained and rinsed
- 1/2 cup diced bell peppers
- 1/4 cup diced onions
- 1/4 cup shredded cheddar cheese
- Salsa for serving

Instructions:

1. Heat a skillet over medium heat and scramble the eggs until cooked through.
2. Warm the tortillas in the skillet or microwave for a few seconds.
3. Divide the scrambled eggs, black beans, bell peppers, onions, and cheese evenly between the tortillas.
4. Roll up the tortillas, tucking in the ends to form burritos.
5. Serve with salsa on the side for dipping.

Nutrition Information:

- Calories: 350
- Protein: 20g
- Carbohydrates: 30g
- Fat: 15g
- Fiber: 8g
- Sugar: 2g
- Portion size: 1 burrito

Quinoa Breakfast Porridge

Ingredients:

- 1/2 cup quinoa, rinsed
- 1 cup almond milk
- 1/2 teaspoon cinnamon
- 1 tablespoon honey or maple syrup
- Fresh fruit for topping (such as sliced bananas or berries)
- Nuts or seeds for topping (such as chopped almonds or pumpkin seeds)

Instructions:

1. In a saucepan, combine quinoa, almond milk, and cinnamon.
2. Bring to a boil, then reduce heat to low and simmer for 15-20 minutes, or until quinoa is cooked and mixture has thickened.
3. Stir in honey or maple syrup.
4. Divide porridge into bowls and top with fresh fruit and nuts or seeds.
5. Serve hot and enjoy!

Nutrition Information:

- Calories: 300
- Protein: 10g
- Carbohydrates: 50g
- Fat: 6g
- Fiber: 6g
- Sugar: 15g
- Portion size: 1 serving

Almond Butter Toast with Banana Slices

Ingredients:

- 2 slices whole grain bread, toasted
- 2 tablespoons almond butter
- 1 banana, sliced

Instructions:

1. Spread almond butter evenly onto each slice of toast.
2. Top with banana slices.
3. Serve immediately and enjoy!

Nutrition Information:

- Calories: 350
- Protein: 10g
- Carbohydrates: 40g
- Fat: 18g
- Fiber: 8g
- Sugar: 15g
- Portion size: 1 serving

Breakfast Muffin Tin Frittatas

Ingredients:

- 6 eggs
- 1/4 cup milk or almond milk
- 1/2 cup diced bell peppers
- 1/2 cup diced onions
- 1/2 cup chopped spinach
- Salt and pepper to taste
- Optional toppings: shredded cheese, cooked bacon or sausage

Instructions:

1. Preheat oven to 350°F (175°C) and lightly grease a muffin tin.
2. In a bowl, whisk together eggs and milk.
3. Stir in diced bell peppers, onions, spinach, salt, and pepper.
4. Pour egg mixture into muffin cups, filling each about 3/4 full.
5. Add optional toppings if desired.
6. Bake for 20-25 minutes, or until frittatas are set and lightly golden.

7. Allow to cool slightly before removing from muffin tin.

8. Serve warm or at room temperature.

Nutrition Information:

- Calories: 150 (per frittata)

- Protein: 10g

- Carbohydrates: 5g

- Fat: 10g

- Fiber: 1g

- Sugar: 2g

- Portion size: 2 frittatas

Smoked Salmon and Cream Cheese Bagel

Ingredients:

- 1 whole grain bagel, sliced and toasted

- 2 tablespoons low-fat cream cheese

- 2 slices smoked salmon

- Thinly sliced red onion (optional)

- Capers for garnish (optional)

- Fresh dill for garnish (optional)

Instructions:

1. Spread cream cheese evenly onto each half of the toasted bagel.
2. Layer smoked salmon on top of the cream cheese.
3. Add thinly sliced red onion, capers, and fresh dill if desired.
4. Serve immediately and enjoy!

Nutrition Information:

- Calories: 350
- Protein: 20g
- Carbohydrates: 40g
- Fat: 12g
- Fiber: 6g
- Sugar: 5g
- Portion size: 1 serving

Cottage Cheese Pancakes

Ingredients:

- 1/2 cup cottage cheese

- 2 eggs
- 1/4 cup almond flour
- 1/4 teaspoon baking powder
- 1/2 teaspoon vanilla extract
- Optional toppings: fresh berries, Greek yogurt, maple syrup

Instructions:

1. In a blender or food processor, combine cottage cheese, eggs, almond flour, baking powder, and vanilla extract.
2. Blend until smooth.
3. Heat a non-stick skillet over medium heat and lightly grease with oil or cooking spray.
4. Pour batter onto the skillet to form pancakes.
5. Cook for 2-3 minutes on each side, or until golden brown.
6. Serve hot with your favorite toppings.

Nutrition Information:
- Calories: 300
- Protein: 25g

- Carbohydrates: 10g

- Fat: 15g

- Fiber: 2g

- Sugar: 5g

- Portion size: 2 pancakes

Tofu Scramble with Veggies

Ingredients:

- 1/2 block firm tofu, crumbled

- 1/2 cup diced bell peppers

- 1/2 cup diced onions

- 1/2 cup chopped spinach

- 1/4 teaspoon turmeric

- Salt and pepper to taste

Instructions:

1. Heat a non-stick skillet over medium heat.

2. Add crumbled tofu, bell peppers, and onions to the skillet.

3. Cook for 5-7 minutes, or until vegetables are tender.

4. Stir in chopped spinach, turmeric, salt, and pepper.

5. Cook for another 2-3 minutes, or until spinach is wilted and tofu is heated through.

6. Serve hot and enjoy!

Nutrition Information:

- Calories: 200
- Protein: 15g
- Carbohydrates: 10g
- Fat: 10g
- Fiber: 4g
- Sugar: 3g
- Portion size: 1 serving

Breakfast Quinoa Bowl with Nuts and Fruit

Ingredients:

- 1/2 cup cooked quinoa
- 1/4 cup mixed nuts (such as almonds, walnuts, and pecans), chopped
- 1/4 cup mixed fresh fruit (such as berries, sliced banana, and diced apple)

- 1 tablespoon honey or maple syrup
- Cinnamon for sprinkling

Instructions:

1. In a bowl, layer cooked quinoa, mixed nuts, and mixed fresh fruit.
2. Drizzle with honey or maple syrup.
3. Sprinkle with cinnamon.
4. Serve immediately and enjoy!

Nutrition Information:

- Calories: 300
- Protein: 10g
- Carbohydrates: 40g
- Fat: 12g
- Fiber: 6g
- Sugar: 15g
- Portion size: 1 serving

Baked Egg Cups with Spinach and Tomatoes

Ingredients:

- 6 eggs
- 1 cup chopped spinach
- 1/2 cup diced tomatoes
- Salt and pepper to taste
- Optional toppings: shredded cheese, cooked bacon or sausage

Instructions:

1. Preheat oven to 350°F (175°C) and lightly grease a muffin tin.
2. Crack an egg into each muffin cup.
3. Divide chopped spinach and diced tomatoes evenly between the muffin cups.
4. Season with salt and pepper.
5. Bake for 15-20 minutes, or until eggs are set.
6. Allow to cool slightly before removing from muffin tin.
7. Serve warm and enjoy!

Nutrition Information:

- Calories: 150 (per egg cup)
- Protein: 10g
- Carbohydrates: 5g
- Fat: 10g
- Fiber: 2g
- Sugar: 2g
- Portion size: 2 egg cups

Zucchini and Bacon Breakfast Hash

Ingredients:

- 2 medium zucchinis, diced
- 4 slices bacon, chopped
- 1/2 cup diced onions
- 1/2 cup diced bell peppers
- 2 cloves garlic, minced
- Salt and pepper to taste
- Optional toppings: fried or poached eggs, avocado slices, hot sauce

Instructions:

1. In a skillet, cook chopped bacon over medium heat until crispy.
2. Remove bacon from skillet and set aside, leaving bacon drippings in the skillet.
3. Add diced zucchinis, onions, bell peppers, and minced garlic to the skillet.
4. Cook, stirring occasionally, until vegetables are tender and slightly browned.
5. Stir in cooked bacon and season with salt and pepper.
6. Serve hot with optional toppings if desired.

Nutrition Information:

- Calories: 300
- Protein: 10g
- Carbohydrates: 10g
- Fat: 20g
- Fiber: 3g
- Sugar: 5g
- Portion size: 1 serving

Chapter 3: Lunch Recipes

In the bustling midday hours, a satisfying lunch can make all the difference in your day. From hearty salads to flavorful wraps, these recipes are designed to keep you fueled and focused until dinner time.

Grilled Chicken Caesar Salad

Ingredients:

- Grilled chicken breast
- Romaine lettuce
- Caesar dressing
- Parmesan cheese
- Croutons

Instructions:

1. Chop grilled chicken and romaine lettuce.
2. Toss lettuce with Caesar dressing.
3. Top with chicken, Parmesan cheese, and croutons.

Nutrition Information (per serving):

- Calories: 350
- Protein: 25g
- Carbohydrates: 10g
- Fat: 20g
- Fiber: 4g
- Sugar: 2g
- Portion size: 1 serving

Turkey and Hummus Wrap

Ingredients:

- Whole wheat tortilla
- Sliced turkey breast
- Hummus
- Lettuce
- Tomato
- Cucumber

Instructions:

1. Spread hummus on tortilla.
2. Layer with turkey, lettuce, tomato, and cucumber.
3. Roll tightly and slice in half.

Nutrition Information (per serving):

- Calories: 280
- Protein: 20g
- Carbohydrates: 25g
- Fat: 10g
- Fiber: 6g
- Sugar: 3g
- Portion size: 1 wrap

Quinoa and Black Bean Salad

Ingredients:

- Cooked quinoa
- Black beans
- Bell peppers
- Red onion
- Cilantro
- Lime juice

Instructions:

1. Mix quinoa, black beans, diced bell peppers, and chopped red onion.
2. Toss with chopped cilantro and lime juice.

Nutrition Information (per serving):

- Calories: 280
- Protein: 12g
- Carbohydrates: 45g
- Fat: 5g
- Fiber: 10g
- Sugar: 2g
- Portion size: 1 cup

Asian Chicken Lettuce Wraps

Ingredients:

- Ground chicken
- Hoisin sauce
- Soy sauce
- Garlic
- Ginger
- Water chestnuts
- Lettuce leaves

Instructions:

1. Brown ground chicken with minced garlic and ginger.

2. Stir in hoisin sauce, soy sauce, and diced water chestnuts.

3. Spoon mixture onto lettuce leaves and wrap.

Nutrition Information (per serving):

- Calories: 220
- Protein: 18g
- Carbohydrates: 10g
- Fat: 10g
- Fiber: 2g
- Sugar: 4g
- Portion size: 2 wraps

Mediterranean Chickpea Salad

Ingredients:

- Chickpeas
- Cherry tomatoes
- Cucumber
- Red onion
- Kalamata olives
- Feta cheese
- Olive oil

- Lemon juice
- Oregano

Instructions:

1. Combine chickpeas, halved cherry tomatoes, diced cucumber, sliced red onion, halved Kalamata olives, and crumbled feta cheese.
2. Drizzle with olive oil and lemon juice.
3. Sprinkle with dried oregano and toss to combine.

Nutrition Information (per serving):

- Calories: 320
- Protein: 10g
- Carbohydrates: 30g
- Fat: 18g
- Fiber: 8g
- Sugar: 5g
- Portion size: 1 cup

Veggie Stir-Fry with Tofu

Ingredients:

- Firm tofu

- Mixed vegetables (bell peppers, broccoli, carrots, snap peas)
- Soy sauce
- Sesame oil
- Garlic
- Ginger
- Green onions

Instructions:

1. Press tofu to remove excess moisture, then cube.
2. Stir-fry tofu in sesame oil with minced garlic and ginger.
3. Add mixed vegetables and soy sauce, cook until tender-crisp.
4. Garnish with sliced green onions.

Nutrition Information (per serving):

- Calories: 240
- Protein: 18g
- Carbohydrates: 15g
- Fat: 12g
- Fiber: 6g

- Sugar: 4g
- Portion size: 1 cup

Tuna Salad Stuffed Avocado

Ingredients:

- Canned tuna
- Avocado
- Red onion
- Celery
- Dijon mustard
- Lemon juice
- Salt and pepper

Instructions:

1. Mix drained canned tuna with diced red onion, diced celery, Dijon mustard, and lemon juice.
2. Cut avocado in half and remove pit.
3. Fill avocado halves with tuna salad mixture.
4. Season with salt and pepper to taste.

Nutrition Information (per serving):

- Calories: 220

- Protein: 15g

- Carbohydrates: 10g

- Fat: 15g

- Fiber: 7g

- Sugar: 2g

- Portion size: 1 stuffed avocado

Caprese Panini with Whole Grain Bread

Ingredients:

- Whole grain bread

- Fresh mozzarella

- Tomato

- Fresh basil

- Balsamic glaze

Instructions:

1. Assemble sandwich with sliced fresh mozzarella, tomato slices, and fresh basil leaves on whole grain bread.

2. Grill in a panini press until bread is toasted and cheese is melted.

3. Drizzle with balsamic glaze before serving.

Nutrition Information (per serving):

- Calories: 280

- Protein: 15g

- Carbohydrates: 30g

- Fat: 12g

- Fiber: 5g

- Sugar: 4g

- Portion size: 1 sandwich

Lentil and Vegetable Soup

Ingredients:

- Lentils

- Carrots

- Celery

- Onion

- Garlic

- Vegetable broth

- Canned diced tomatoes

- Bay leaf
- Thyme
- Salt and pepper

Instructions:

1. Sauté diced onion, carrots, and celery until softened.
2. Add minced garlic and cook for another minute.
3. Stir in lentils, vegetable broth, canned diced tomatoes, bay leaf, and thyme.
4. Simmer until lentils are tender, then season with salt and pepper to taste.

Nutrition Information (per serving):

- Calories: 220
- Protein: 12g
- Carbohydrates: 40g
- Fat: 2g
- Fiber: 12g
- Sugar: 6g
- Portion size: 1 cup

Shrimp and Quinoa Salad

Ingredients:

- Cooked shrimp
- Cooked quinoa
- Bell peppers
- Cucumber
- Cherry tomatoes
- Red onion
- Lemon vinaigrette
- Fresh parsley

Instructions:

1. Combine cooked shrimp, cooked quinoa, diced bell peppers, diced cucumber, halved cherry tomatoes, and thinly sliced red onion.
2. Toss with lemon vinaigrette and chopped fresh parsley.

Nutrition Information (per serving):

- Calories: 280
- Protein: 20g
- Carbohydrates: 25g

- Fat: 10g

- Fiber: 6g

- Sugar: 3g

- Portion size: 1 cup

Chicken and Veggie Kebabs

Ingredients:

- Chicken breast

- Bell peppers

- Zucchini

- Red onion

- Olive oil

- Garlic powder

- Paprika

- Salt and pepper

Instructions:

1. Cut chicken breast into chunks and chop bell peppers, zucchini, and red onion into bite-sized pieces.

2. Thread chicken and veggies onto skewers.

3. Brush with olive oil and sprinkle with garlic powder, paprika, salt, and pepper.

4. Grill until chicken is cooked through and veggies are tender.

Nutrition Information (per serving):

- Calories: 250
- Protein: 30g
- Carbohydrates: 10g
- Fat: 10g
- Fiber: 3g
- Sugar: 5g
- Portion size: 1 skewer

Egg Salad Lettuce Wraps

Ingredients:

- Hard-boiled eggs
- Greek yogurt
- Dijon mustard
- Green onions
- Dill
- Salt and pepper

- Lettuce leaves

Instructions:

1. Chop hard-boiled eggs and mix with Greek yogurt, Dijon mustard, chopped green onions, dill, salt, and pepper.
2. Spoon egg salad onto lettuce leaves.
3. Roll lettuce leaves to form wraps.

Nutrition Information (per serving):

- Calories: 180
- Protein: 15g
- Carbohydrates: 5g
- Fat: 10g
- Fiber: 2g
- Sugar: 2g
- Portion size: 2 wraps

Turkey and Vegetable Skewers

Ingredients:

- Turkey breast
- Bell peppers

- Cherry tomatoes
- Red onion
- Olive oil
- Italian seasoning
- Salt and pepper

Instructions:

1. Cut turkey breast into chunks and chop bell peppers and red onion into bite-sized pieces.
2. Thread turkey and veggies onto skewers.
3. Brush with olive oil and sprinkle with Italian seasoning, salt, and pepper.
4. Grill until turkey is cooked through and veggies are tender.

Nutrition Information (per serving):

- Calories: 220
- Protein: 25g
- Carbohydrates: 10g
- Fat: 8g
- Fiber: 3g
- Sugar: 5g
- Portion size: 1 skewer

Greek Salad with Grilled Halloumi

Ingredients:

- Romaine lettuce
- Cucumber
- Cherry tomatoes
- Kalamata olives
- Red onion
- Grilled halloumi cheese
- Olive oil
- Red wine vinegar
- Dried oregano
- Salt and pepper

Instructions:

1. Chop romaine lettuce and dice cucumber, halve cherry tomatoes, slice red onion, and cube grilled halloumi cheese.
2. Combine all ingredients in a bowl.
3. Drizzle with olive oil and red wine vinegar.
4. Season with dried oregano, salt, and pepper.

Nutrition Information (per serving):

- Calories: 320
- Protein: 15g
- Carbohydrates: 15g
- Fat: 22g
- Fiber: 6g
- Sugar: 5g
- Portion size: 1.5 cups

Cauliflower Crust Pizza with Salad

Ingredients:

- Cauliflower
- Mozzarella cheese
- Parmesan cheese
- Egg
- Tomato sauce
- Italian seasoning
- Toppings of choice (e.g., bell peppers, mushrooms, onions)
- Mixed greens
- Balsamic vinaigrette

Instructions:

1. Rice cauliflower in a food processor and steam until tender. Let cool.
2. Mix cauliflower with shredded mozzarella cheese, grated Parmesan cheese, and beaten egg to form a dough.
3. Press dough onto a baking sheet lined with parchment paper to form a crust.
4. Bake crust in preheated oven until golden brown.
5. Spread tomato sauce over crust, sprinkle with Italian seasoning, and add desired toppings.
6. Return to oven and bake until toppings are heated through.
7. Serve pizza with a side of mixed greens tossed in balsamic vinaigrette.

Nutrition Information (per serving):

- Calories: 280
- Protein: 15g
- Carbohydrates: 15g
- Fat: 18g
- Fiber: 5g

- Sugar: 4g
- Portion size: 1/4 pizza with salad

Chapter 4: Dinner Recipes

These dishes are crafted to satisfy your taste buds while also supporting your health goals, particularly for managing type 1 diabetes. From succulent seafood to hearty meat options and vibrant vegetarian fare, there's something here to suit every palate.

Baked Salmon with Asparagus

Ingredients:

- 4 salmon fillets
- 1 bunch asparagus, trimmed
- Olive oil
- Salt and pepper
- Lemon slices
- Fresh dill (optional)

Instructions:

1. Preheat the oven to 400°F (200°C).
2. Place salmon fillets and asparagus on a baking sheet.

3. Drizzle with olive oil and season with salt and pepper.

4. Arrange lemon slices over the salmon.

5. Bake for 12-15 minutes, or until salmon is cooked through and asparagus is tender.

6. Garnish with fresh dill before serving.

Nutrition Information (per serving):

- Calories: 320

- Protein: 30g

- Carbohydrates: 5g

- Fat: 20g

- Fiber: 2g

- Sugar: 2g

- Portion size: 1 fillet with asparagus

Spaghetti Squash with Turkey Bolognese

Ingredients:

- 1 spaghetti squash

- 1 lb ground turkey

- 1 onion, diced

- 2 cloves garlic, minced

- 1 can (14 oz) crushed tomatoes

- Italian seasoning

- Salt and pepper

- Fresh parsley, chopped (for garnish)

Instructions:

1. Preheat the oven to 375°F (190°C).

2. Cut the spaghetti squash in half lengthwise and remove the seeds.

3. Place squash halves, cut side down, on a baking sheet.

4. Bake for 30-40 minutes, or until squash is tender.

5. In a skillet, brown ground turkey with onion and garlic.

6. Add crushed tomatoes and season with Italian seasoning, salt, and pepper.

7. Simmer for 10-15 minutes.

8. Use a fork to scrape the spaghetti squash into strands.

9. Serve turkey bolognese over spaghetti squash.

10. Garnish with chopped parsley.

Nutrition Information (per serving):

- Calories: 280
- Protein: 25g
- Carbohydrates: 20g
- Fat: 12g
- Fiber: 5g
- Sugar: 8g
- Portion size: 1 cup squash with turkey bolognese

Lemon Garlic Chicken with Roasted Vegetables

Ingredients:

- 4 boneless, skinless chicken breasts
- 2 cups mixed vegetables (such as carrots, bell peppers, and broccoli)
- 2 tablespoons olive oil
- 2 cloves garlic, minced
- 1 lemon, juiced and zested
- Salt and pepper
- Fresh parsley, chopped (for garnish)

Instructions:

1. Preheat the oven to 400°F (200°C).
2. Place chicken breasts and mixed vegetables on a baking sheet.
3. In a small bowl, whisk together olive oil, minced garlic, lemon juice, and lemon zest.
4. Drizzle the lemon garlic mixture over the chicken and vegetables.
5. Season with salt and pepper.
6. Bake for 20-25 minutes, or until chicken is cooked through and vegetables are tender.
7. Garnish with chopped parsley before serving.

Nutrition Information (per serving):

- Calories: 280
- Protein: 30g
- Carbohydrates: 10g
- Fat: 12g
- Fiber: 3g
- Sugar: 4g
- Portion size: 1 chicken breast with vegetables

Cauliflower Fried Rice with Shrimp

Ingredients:

- 1 head cauliflower, grated
- 1 lb shrimp, peeled and deveined
- 2 eggs, beaten
- 1 cup mixed vegetables (such as peas, carrots, and green onions)
- 2 tablespoons soy sauce (or tamari for gluten-free)
- 1 tablespoon sesame oil
- 2 cloves garlic, minced
- Salt and pepper
- Green onions, sliced (for garnish)

Instructions:

1. In a large skillet, heat sesame oil over medium heat.
2. Add minced garlic and cook until fragrant.
3. Add shrimp and cook until pink and opaque, about 2-3 minutes per side.
4. Push shrimp to one side of the skillet and pour beaten eggs into the other side.
5. Scramble eggs until cooked through, then mix with shrimp.

6. Add grated cauliflower and mixed vegetables to the skillet.

7. Stir in soy sauce and season with salt and pepper to taste.

8. Cook until cauliflower is tender, about 5-7 minutes.

9. Garnish with sliced green onions before serving.

Nutrition Information (per serving):

- Calories: 250

- Protein: 25g

- Carbohydrates: 15g

- Fat: 10g

- Fiber: 5g

- Sugar: 5g

- Portion size: 1 cup of cauliflower fried rice with shrimp

Stuffed Bell Peppers with Ground Turkey

Ingredients:

- 4 bell peppers, halved and seeds removed

- 1 lb lean ground turkey

- 1 onion, diced

- 2 cloves garlic, minced

- 1 cup cooked quinoa

- 1 can (14 oz) diced tomatoes

- 1 teaspoon Italian seasoning

- Salt and pepper

- Fresh parsley, chopped (for garnish)

Instructions:

1. Preheat the oven to 375°F (190°C).

2. In a skillet, brown ground turkey with diced onion and minced garlic.

3. Stir in cooked quinoa, diced tomatoes, and Italian seasoning.

4. Season with salt and pepper to taste.

5. Place bell pepper halves in a baking dish.

6. Spoon turkey and quinoa mixture into each pepper half.

7. Cover the dish with foil and bake for 25-30 minutes.

8. Remove foil and bake for an additional 10 minutes, or until peppers are tender.

9. Garnish with chopped parsley before serving.

Nutrition Information (per serving):

- Calories: 280
- Protein: 25g
- Carbohydrates: 20g
- Fat: 10g
- Fiber: 5g
- Sugar: 8g
- Portion size: 1 stuffed bell pepper half

Beef and Broccoli Stir-Fry

Ingredients:

- 1 lb flank steak, thinly sliced
- 2 cups broccoli florets
- 1 bell pepper, sliced
- 2 cloves garlic, minced
- 1 tablespoon ginger, minced
- 1/4 cup low-sodium soy sauce (or tamari for gluten-free)
- 2 tablespoons oyster sauce
- 1 tablespoon sesame oil

- 1 tablespoon cornstarch
- 2 tablespoons water
- Cooked brown rice, for serving
- Sesame seeds, for garnish

Instructions:

1. In a small bowl, whisk together soy sauce, oyster sauce, sesame oil, cornstarch, and water to make the sauce.
2. Heat a tablespoon of oil in a large skillet or wok over medium-high heat.
3. Add sliced flank steak and stir-fry until browned, about 2-3 minutes.
4. Remove steak from the skillet and set aside.
5. In the same skillet, add a little more oil if needed, then add minced garlic and ginger. Stir-fry for about 30 seconds until fragrant.
6. Add broccoli florets and sliced bell pepper to the skillet. Stir-fry for about 3-4 minutes until vegetables are crisp-tender.
7. Return the cooked steak to the skillet and pour the sauce over the beef and vegetables.

8. Stir-fry everything together for another 2-3 minutes until the sauce thickens and coats the ingredients.

9. Serve hot over cooked brown rice and garnish with sesame seeds.

Nutrition Information (per serving):

- Calories: 350
- Protein: 30g
- Carbohydrates: 20g
- Fat: 15g
- Fiber: 4g
- Sugar: 4g
- Portion size: 1 cup of beef and broccoli stir-fry with rice

Veggie and Bean Chili

Ingredients:

- 1 tablespoon olive oil
- 1 onion, diced
- 2 cloves garlic, minced
- 1 bell pepper, diced
- 1 zucchini, diced

- 1 carrot, diced

- 1 can (14 oz) diced tomatoes

- 1 can (14 oz) kidney beans, drained and rinsed

- 1 can (14 oz) black beans, drained and rinsed

- 2 cups vegetable broth

- 2 tablespoons chili powder

- 1 teaspoon cumin

- Salt and pepper

- Fresh cilantro, chopped (for garnish)

- Greek yogurt (optional, for serving)

Instructions:

1. Heat olive oil in a large pot over medium heat.

2. Add diced onion and minced garlic, and sauté until softened, about 2-3 minutes.

3. Add diced bell pepper, zucchini, and carrot to the pot, and cook for another 5 minutes until vegetables are tender.

4. Stir in diced tomatoes, kidney beans, black beans, vegetable broth, chili powder, cumin, salt, and pepper.

5. Bring the chili to a boil, then reduce the heat and simmer for 20-25 minutes, stirring occasionally.

6. Adjust seasoning to taste with salt and pepper.

7. Serve hot, garnished with chopped cilantro and a dollop of Greek yogurt if desired.

Nutrition Information (per serving):

- Calories: 280

- Protein: 15g

- Carbohydrates: 45g

- Fat: 5g

- Fiber: 15g

- Sugar: 10g

- Portion size: 1 cup of veggie and bean chili

Grilled Swordfish with Mango Salsa

Ingredients:

- 4 swordfish steaks

- 2 ripe mangoes, diced

- 1 red bell pepper, diced

- 1/4 cup red onion, finely chopped

- 1 jalapeño, seeded and minced

- Juice of 1 lime
- 2 tablespoons fresh cilantro, chopped
- Salt and pepper
- Olive oil

Instructions:

1. Preheat grill to medium-high heat.
2. Season swordfish steaks with salt, pepper, and a drizzle of olive oil.
3. Grill swordfish for 4-5 minutes on each side, or until cooked through and grill marks appear.
4. In a bowl, combine diced mangoes, red bell pepper, red onion, jalapeño, lime juice, and cilantro. Season with salt and pepper to taste.
5. Serve grilled swordfish topped with mango salsa.

Nutrition Information (per serving):

- Calories: 320
- Protein: 30g
- Carbohydrates: 20g
- Fat: 12g
- Fiber: 3g

- Sugar: 15g
- Portion size: 1 swordfish steak with salsa

Zucchini Noodles with Pesto and Grilled Chicken

Ingredients:

- 2 large zucchinis, spiralized into noodles
- 2 boneless, skinless chicken breasts
- 1/2 cup basil pesto
- Cherry tomatoes, halved
- Parmesan cheese, grated (optional)
- Salt and pepper
- Olive oil

Instructions:

1. Preheat grill to medium-high heat.
2. Season chicken breasts with salt, pepper, and a drizzle of olive oil.
3. Grill chicken for 6-8 minutes on each side, or until cooked through.

4. While the chicken is cooking, heat olive oil in a skillet over medium heat.

5. Add zucchini noodles to the skillet and cook for 2-3 minutes until just tender.

6. Remove zucchini noodles from heat and toss with basil pesto.

7. Slice grilled chicken breasts.

8. Serve zucchini noodles topped with sliced chicken, cherry tomatoes, and grated Parmesan cheese if desired.

Nutrition Information (per serving):

- Calories: 350
- Protein: 30g
- Carbohydrates: 10g
- Fat: 20g
- Fiber: 3g
- Sugar: 5g
- Portion size: 1 chicken breast with zucchini noodles

Pork Tenderloin with Roasted Brussels Sprouts

Ingredients:

- 1 lb pork tenderloin
- 1 lb Brussels sprouts, halved
- 2 tablespoons olive oil
- 2 cloves garlic, minced
- 1 teaspoon dried thyme
- Salt and pepper

Instructions:

1. Preheat the oven to 400°F (200°C).
2. Place pork tenderloin and Brussels sprouts on a baking sheet.
3. In a small bowl, mix together olive oil, minced garlic, dried thyme, salt, and pepper.
4. Drizzle the olive oil mixture over the pork and Brussels sprouts, ensuring they are evenly coated.
5. Roast in the oven for 25-30 minutes, or until the pork is cooked through and the Brussels sprouts are caramelized.
6. Let the pork rest for a few minutes before slicing.

7. Serve the pork tenderloin with roasted Brussels sprouts.

Nutrition Information (per serving):

- Calories: 280
- Protein: 25g
- Carbohydrates: 10g
- Fat: 15g
- Fiber: 5g
- Sugar: 3g
- Portion size: 1/4 of the pork tenderloin with Brussels sprouts

Turkey Meatballs with Marinara Sauce

Ingredients:

- 1 lb lean ground turkey
- 1/2 cup breadcrumbs (whole wheat or gluten-free)
- 1/4 cup grated Parmesan cheese
- 1 egg
- 2 cloves garlic, minced

- 1 teaspoon dried oregano

- 1/2 teaspoon dried basil

- Salt and pepper

- 2 cups marinara sauce

- Fresh parsley, chopped (for garnish)

Instructions:

1. Preheat the oven to 400°F (200°C).

2. In a large bowl, combine ground turkey, breadcrumbs, Parmesan cheese, egg, minced garlic, dried oregano, dried basil, salt, and pepper.

3. Mix until well combined, then form the mixture into meatballs.

4. Place meatballs on a baking sheet lined with parchment paper.

5. Bake in the preheated oven for 20-25 minutes, or until cooked through.

6. In a saucepan, heat marinara sauce over medium heat.

7. Add cooked meatballs to the marinara sauce and simmer for a few minutes.

8. Serve hot, garnished with chopped parsley.

Nutrition Information (per serving):

- Calories: 250

- Protein: 20g

- Carbohydrates: 10g

- Fat: 12g

- Fiber: 2g

- Sugar: 5g

- Portion size: 4 meatballs with sauce

Ratatouille with Quinoa

Ingredients:

- 1 eggplant, diced

- 2 zucchinis, diced

- 1 bell pepper, diced

- 1 onion, diced

- 2 cloves garlic, minced

- 2 tomatoes, diced

- 1 can (14 oz) tomato sauce

- 1 teaspoon dried thyme

- 1 teaspoon dried basil

- Salt and pepper

- Cooked quinoa, for serving

- Fresh basil, chopped (for garnish)

Instructions:

1. Heat olive oil in a large pot over medium heat.

2. Add diced onion and minced garlic, and sauté until softened, about 2-3 minutes.

3. Add diced eggplant, zucchini, bell pepper, and tomatoes to the pot.

4. Stir in tomato sauce, dried thyme, dried basil, salt, and pepper.

5. Cover and simmer for 20-25 minutes, stirring occasionally, until vegetables are tender.

6. Serve ratatouille over cooked quinoa.

7. Garnish with chopped fresh basil before serving.

Nutrition Information (per serving):

- Calories: 280

- Protein: 8g

- Carbohydrates: 45g

- Fat: 5g

- Fiber: 12g

- Sugar: 12g

- Portion size: 1 cup of ratatouille with quinoa

Chicken Curry with Cauliflower Rice

Ingredients:

- 1 lb boneless, skinless chicken thighs, cut into bite-sized pieces
- 1 onion, diced
- 2 cloves garlic, minced
- 1 bell pepper, sliced
- 1 cup coconut milk
- 1 can (14 oz) diced tomatoes
- 2 tablespoons curry powder
- 1 teaspoon turmeric
- Salt and pepper
- Fresh cilantro, chopped (for garnish)
- Cauliflower rice, for serving

Instructions:

1. Heat olive oil in a large skillet over medium heat.
2. Add diced onion and minced garlic, and sauté until softened, about 2-3 minutes.

3. Add sliced bell pepper and cook for another 2 minutes.

4. Add chicken pieces to the skillet and cook until browned on all sides.

5. Stir in coconut milk, diced tomatoes, curry powder, turmeric, salt, and pepper.

6. Cover and simmer for 15-20 minutes, until chicken is cooked through and sauce is thickened.

7. Serve chicken curry over cauliflower rice.

8. Garnish with chopped fresh cilantro before serving.

Nutrition Information (per serving):

- Calories: 350

- Protein: 25g

- Carbohydrates: 15g

- Fat: 20g

- Fiber: 5g

- Sugar: 8g

- Portion size: 1 cup of chicken curry with cauliflower rice

Beef Stir-Fry with Ginger and Snap Peas

Ingredients:

- 1 lb beef sirloin, thinly sliced
- 2 cups snap peas
- 1 bell pepper, sliced
- 1 onion, sliced
- 2 cloves garlic, minced
- 1 tablespoon fresh ginger, minced
- 3 tablespoons low-sodium soy sauce (or tamari for gluten-free)
- 1 tablespoon rice vinegar
- 1 tablespoon sesame oil
- 1 teaspoon cornstarch
- 2 tablespoons water
- Cooked brown rice, for serving
- Sesame seeds, for garnish

Instructions:

1. In a small bowl, mix together soy sauce, rice vinegar, sesame oil, cornstarch, and water to make the sauce.

2. Heat a tablespoon of oil in a large skillet or wok over medium-high heat.

3. Add sliced beef and stir-fry until browned, about 2-3 minutes.

4. Remove beef from the skillet and set aside.

5. In the same skillet, add a little more oil if needed, then add minced garlic and minced ginger. Stir-fry for about 30 seconds until fragrant.

6. Add snap peas, sliced bell pepper, and sliced onion to the skillet. Stir-fry for about 3-4 minutes until vegetables are crisp-tender.

7. Return the cooked beef to the skillet and pour the sauce over the beef and vegetables.

8. Stir-fry everything together for another 2-3 minutes until the sauce thickens and coats the ingredients.

9. Serve hot over cooked brown rice and garnish with sesame seeds.

Nutrition Information (per serving):

- Calories: 320

- Protein: 25g

- Carbohydrates: 20g

- Fat: 15g

- Fiber: 4g

- Sugar: 8g

- Portion size: 1 cup of beef stir-fry with rice

Baked Cod with Herbed Quinoa

Ingredients:

- 4 cod fillets

- 1 cup quinoa, rinsed

- 2 cups vegetable broth

- 2 cloves garlic, minced

- 2 tablespoons fresh herbs (such as parsley, dill, or chives), chopped

- 1 lemon, juiced and zested

- Salt and pepper

- Olive oil

Instructions:

1. Preheat the oven to 400°F (200°C).

2. In a saucepan, bring vegetable broth to a boil.

3. Add rinsed quinoa and minced garlic to the saucepan. Reduce heat, cover, and simmer for 15-20 minutes until quinoa is cooked and liquid is absorbed.

4. Fluff the quinoa with a fork and stir in chopped fresh herbs, lemon juice, and lemon zest. Season with salt and pepper to taste.

5. Place cod fillets on a baking sheet lined with parchment paper.

6. Drizzle cod fillets with olive oil and season with salt and pepper.

7. Bake in the preheated oven for 12-15 minutes, or until cod is cooked through and flakes easily with a fork.

8. Serve baked cod over herbed quinoa.

Nutrition Information (per serving):

- Calories: 300
- Protein: 25g
- Carbohydrates: 30g
- Fat: 10g
- Fiber: 4g
- Sugar: 2g
- Portion size: 1 cod fillet with quinoa

Chapter 5: Snacks and Appetizers

In this chapter, we'll explore a variety of snacks and appetizers that are not only satisfying but also suitable for managing your blood sugar levels. From crunchy veggies paired with creamy dips to protein-packed bites, these snacks will keep you fueled throughout the day.

Veggie Sticks with Hummus

Ingredients:

- Assorted fresh vegetables (carrots, celery, bell peppers, cucumber)
- Hummus

Instructions:

1. Wash and cut the vegetables into sticks.
2. Serve with a side of hummus for dipping.

Nutrition Information (per serving):

- Calories: 100
- Protein: 4g

- Carbohydrates: 12g

- Fat: 5g

- Fiber: 4g

- Sugar: 3g

- Portion size: 1 cup of veggies with 2 tbsp hummus

Greek Yogurt Dip with Fresh Veggies

Ingredients:

- Greek yogurt

- Assorted fresh vegetables (cherry tomatoes, cucumber, bell peppers)

Instructions:

1. Mix Greek yogurt with your favorite herbs and spices.

2. Serve with fresh vegetable sticks for dipping.

Nutrition Information (per serving):

- Calories: 80

- Protein: 6g

- Carbohydrates: 8g

- Fat: 3g

- Fiber: 2g

- Sugar: 4g

- Portion size: 1/2 cup Greek yogurt with 1 cup of veggies

Apple Slices with Almond Butter

Ingredients:

- Apple

- Almond butter

Instructions:

1. Slice the apple into wedges.

2. Spread almond butter on each apple slice.

Nutrition Information (per serving):

- Calories: 150

- Protein: 4g

- Carbohydrates: 15g

- Fat: 9g

- Fiber: 4g

- Sugar: 10g
- Portion size: 1 medium apple with 2 tbsp almond butter

Cheese and Whole Grain Crackers

Ingredients:
- Cheese slices or cubes
- Whole grain crackers

Instructions:
1. Place cheese on top of whole grain crackers.

Nutrition Information (per serving):
- Calories: 120
- Protein: 6g
- Carbohydrates: 10g
- Fat: 6g
- Fiber: 2g
- Sugar: 1g
- Portion size: 1 ounce cheese with 5 crackers

Hard-Boiled Eggs with Mustard

Ingredients:

- Hard-boiled eggs
- Mustard

Instructions:

1. Peel hard-boiled eggs.
2. Serve with a dollop of mustard on the side.

Nutrition Information (per serving):

- Calories: 70
- Protein: 6g
- Carbohydrates: 1g
- Fat: 5g
- Fiber: 0g
- Sugar: 0g
- Portion size: 2 hard-boiled eggs with 1 tbsp mustard

Mixed Nuts and Seeds

Ingredients:

- Assorted nuts (almonds, walnuts, cashews)

- Assorted seeds (pumpkin seeds, sunflower seeds)

Instructions:

1. Mix nuts and seeds together in a bowl.

2. Portion out a small handful for a snack.

Nutrition Information (per serving):

- Calories: 180

- Protein: 7g

- Carbohydrates: 5g

- Fat: 15g

- Fiber: 3g

- Sugar: 1g

- Portion size: 1/4 cup mixed nuts and seeds

Edamame with Sea Salt

Ingredients:

- Edamame (fresh or frozen)

- Sea salt

Instructions:

1. Cook edamame according to package instructions.

2. Sprinkle with sea salt before serving.

Nutrition Information (per serving):

- Calories: 100

- Protein: 9g

- Carbohydrates: 9g

- Fat: 3g

- Fiber: 5g

- Sugar: 2g

- Portion size: 1 cup edamame

Cucumber Slices with Cream Cheese

Ingredients:

- Cucumber

- Cream cheese

Instructions:

1. Slice cucumber into rounds.
2. Spread cream cheese on each cucumber slice.

Nutrition Information (per serving):

- Calories: 70

- Protein: 2g

- Carbohydrates: 3g

- Fat: 5g

- Fiber: 1g

- Sugar: 2g

- Portion size: 1 medium cucumber with 2 tbsp cream cheese

Baked Kale Chips

Ingredients:

- Fresh kale leaves

- Olive oil

- Salt

Instructions:

1. Preheat oven to 350°F (175°C).

2. Remove stems from kale leaves and tear into bite-sized pieces.

3. Toss kale with olive oil and a pinch of salt.

4. Spread kale evenly on a baking sheet.

5. Bake for 10-15 minutes until crisp.

6. Allow to cool before serving.

Nutrition Information (per serving):

- Calories: 50
- Protein: 2g
- Carbohydrates: 4g
- Fat: 3g
- Fiber: 1g
- Sugar: 0g
- Portion size: 1 cup kale chips

Cottage Cheese with Pineapple Chunks

Ingredients:

- Cottage cheese
- Fresh pineapple chunks

Instructions:

1. Spoon cottage cheese into a bowl.
2. Top with pineapple chunks.

Nutrition Information (per serving):

- Calories: 120

- Protein: 15g

- Carbohydrates: 10g

- Fat: 2g

- Fiber: 1g

- Sugar: 8g

- Portion size: 1/2 cup cottage cheese with 1/2 cup pineapple chunks

Mini Caprese Skewers

Ingredients:

- Cherry tomatoes

- Fresh mozzarella balls

- Fresh basil leaves

- Balsamic glaze (optional)

Instructions:

1. Thread a cherry tomato, a mozzarella ball, and a basil leaf onto a toothpick or skewer.

2. Repeat with remaining ingredients.

3. Drizzle with balsamic glaze if desired before serving.

Nutrition Information (per serving):

- Calories: 80
- Protein: 5g
- Carbohydrates: 3g
- Fat: 6g
- Fiber: 1g
- Sugar: 2g
- Portion size: 4 skewers

Roasted Chickpeas

Ingredients:

- Canned chickpeas (garbanzo beans)
- Olive oil
- Seasonings (such as garlic powder, paprika, cumin)
- Salt

Instructions:

1. Preheat oven to 400°F (200°C).
2. Rinse and drain chickpeas, then pat dry with a paper towel.
3. Toss chickpeas with olive oil, seasonings, and salt.
4. Spread chickpeas in a single layer on a baking sheet.

5. Roast for 20-30 minutes, shaking the pan occasionally, until crispy.

6. Allow to cool before serving.

Nutrition Information (per serving):

- Calories: 120

- Protein: 5g

- Carbohydrates: 16g

- Fat: 4g

- Fiber: 5g

- Sugar: 3g

- Portion size: 1/2 cup roasted chickpeas

Turkey and Cheese Roll-Ups

Ingredients:

- Deli turkey slices

- Cheese slices (cheddar, Swiss, or your choice)

- Mustard or mayonnaise (optional)

Instructions:

1. Lay turkey slices flat on a clean surface.

2. Place a cheese slice on top of each turkey slice.

3. Add a small amount of mustard or mayonnaise if desired.

4. Roll up tightly and secure with toothpicks if necessary.

Nutrition Information (per serving):

- Calories: 120
- Protein: 12g
- Carbohydrates: 1g
- Fat: 8g
- Fiber: 0g
- Sugar: 0g
- Portion size: 2 roll-ups

Avocado Salsa with Baked Tortilla Chips

Ingredients:

- Avocado
- Tomato
- Onion
- Cilantro

- Lime juice

- Salt

- Baked tortilla chips

Instructions:

1. Dice avocado, tomato, onion, and cilantro.

2. Mix together in a bowl with lime juice and salt to taste.

3. Serve with baked tortilla chips.

Nutrition Information (per serving):

- Calories: 150

- Protein: 2g

- Carbohydrates: 10g

- Fat: 12g

- Fiber: 5g

- Sugar: 2g

- Portion size: 1/2 cup avocado salsa with 1 serving of tortilla chips

Stuffed Mushrooms with Spinach and Feta

Ingredients:

- Large mushrooms
- Spinach
- Feta cheese
- Garlic
- Olive oil
- Salt and pepper

Instructions:

1. Preheat oven to 375°F (190°C).
2. Remove stems from mushrooms and chop finely.
3. Sauté chopped mushroom stems, spinach, garlic, and a dash of salt and pepper in olive oil until wilted.
4. Stuff mushroom caps with spinach mixture and top with crumbled feta cheese.
5. Bake for 15-20 minutes until mushrooms are tender and cheese is melted.

Nutrition Information (per serving):

- Calories: 80

- Protein: 5g

- Carbohydrates: 5g

- Fat: 5g

- Fiber: 2g

- Sugar: 2g

- Portion size: 2 stuffed mushrooms

Chapter 6: Desserts

This chapter is filled with fifteen delightful dessert recipes crafted with wholesome ingredients and mindful portions to satisfy your sweet tooth while keeping your blood sugar levels in check. From refreshing fruit popsicles to decadent chocolate treats, each recipe offers a balance of flavors and nutrients to support your well-being.

Berry and Yogurt Popsicles

Ingredients:

- 1 cup mixed berries (such as strawberries, blueberries, raspberries)
- 1 cup plain Greek yogurt
- 1 tablespoon honey or maple syrup (optional)

Instructions:

1. Blend the mixed berries until smooth.
2. In a separate bowl, mix the Greek yogurt with honey or maple syrup, if using.

3. Layer the berry puree and yogurt mixture into popsicle molds.

4. Insert popsicle sticks and freeze for at least 4 hours or until firm.

5. Enjoy these refreshing popsicles as a guilt-free dessert option.

Nutrition Information (per serving, makes 4 popsicles):

- Calories: 80
- Protein: 6g
- Carbohydrates: 12g
- Fat: 0.5g
- Fiber: 2g
- Sugar: 8g
- Portion size: 1 popsicle

Dark Chocolate Covered Strawberries

Ingredients:

- 1 cup fresh strawberries, washed and dried
- 2 ounces dark chocolate, melted

Instructions:

1. Dip each strawberry into the melted dark chocolate, coating about three-quarters of the berry.
2. Place the chocolate-covered strawberries on a parchment-lined baking sheet.
3. Allow the chocolate to set at room temperature or in the refrigerator.
4. Serve these elegant treats as a delightful dessert or special occasion indulgence.

Nutrition Information (per serving, makes 4 strawberries):

- Calories: 60
- Protein: 1g
- Carbohydrates: 8g
- Fat: 4g
- Fiber: 2g
- Sugar: 4g
- Portion size: 4 strawberries

Sugar-Free Cheesecake Bites

Ingredients:

- 8 ounces cream cheese, softened

- 1/4 cup powdered erythritol or stevia blend

- 1 teaspoon vanilla extract

- Fresh berries for garnish (optional)

Instructions:

1. In a mixing bowl, beat the softened cream cheese until smooth.

2. Add the powdered erythritol or stevia blend and vanilla extract, and mix until well combined.

3. Roll the mixture into small balls and place them on a parchment-lined baking sheet.

4. Chill the cheesecake bites in the refrigerator for at least 1 hour or until firm.

5. Garnish with fresh berries, if desired, before serving.

Nutrition Information (per serving, makes 12 bites):

- Calories: 70

- Protein: 2g

- Carbohydrates: 2g

- Fat: 6g

- Fiber: 0g

- Sugar: 1g

- Portion size: 2 bites

Almond Flour Chocolate Chip Cookies

Ingredients:

- 1 1/2 cups almond flour
- 1/4 cup coconut oil, melted
- 1/4 cup sugar-free chocolate chips
- 1/4 cup powdered erythritol or stevia blend
- 1 egg
- 1 teaspoon vanilla extract

Instructions:

1. Preheat the oven to 350°F (175°C) and line a baking sheet with parchment paper.
2. In a mixing bowl, combine the almond flour, melted coconut oil, sugar-free chocolate chips, powdered erythritol or stevia blend, egg, and vanilla extract. Mix until a dough forms.
3. Roll the dough into balls and place them on the prepared baking sheet.

4. Flatten each ball with the palm of your hand to form cookies.

5. Bake for 10-12 minutes or until the edges are golden brown.

6. Allow the cookies to cool on the baking sheet before serving.

Nutrition Information (per serving, makes 12 cookies):

- Calories: 120

- Protein: 3g

- Carbohydrates: 4g

- Fat: 10g

- Fiber: 1g

- Sugar: 1g

- Portion size: 1 cookie

Greek Yogurt with Honey and Almonds

Ingredients:

- 1 cup plain Greek yogurt

- 1 tablespoon honey

- 2 tablespoons sliced almonds

Instructions:

1. Spoon the Greek yogurt into a serving bowl.
2. Drizzle honey over the yogurt.
3. Sprinkle sliced almonds on top.
4. Serve immediately as a simple and satisfying dessert or snack.

Nutrition Information (per serving):

- Calories: 150
- Protein: 10g
- Carbohydrates: 13g
- Fat: 7g
- Fiber: 1g
- Sugar: 11g
- Portion size: 1 serving

Chia Seed Pudding with Berries

Ingredients:

- 1/4 cup chia seeds
- 1 cup unsweetened almond milk

- 1 tablespoon honey or maple syrup
- 1/2 cup mixed berries (such as strawberries, blueberries, raspberries)

Instructions:

1. In a bowl, combine the chia seeds, almond milk, and honey or maple syrup. Stir well.
2. Let the mixture sit for 5 minutes, then stir again to prevent clumping.
3. Cover the bowl and refrigerate for at least 2 hours or overnight, until the pudding has thickened.
4. Serve the chia seed pudding topped with mixed berries for a nutritious and delicious dessert option.

Nutrition Information (per serving):

- Calories: 140
- Protein: 4g
- Carbohydrates: 18g
- Fat: 6g
- Fiber: 9g
- Sugar: 7g
- Portion size: 1 serving

Baked Apple Slices with Cinnamon

Ingredients:

- 2 apples, cored and sliced
- 1 teaspoon cinnamon
- 1 tablespoon lemon juice
- Stevia or erythritol (optional, to taste)

Instructions:

1. Preheat the oven to 350°F (175°C).
2. In a bowl, toss the apple slices with cinnamon and lemon juice.
3. Arrange the apple slices in a single layer on a baking sheet lined with parchment paper.
4. If desired, sprinkle stevia or erythritol over the apple slices for added sweetness.
5. Bake for 15-20 minutes or until the apples are tender.
6. Serve warm as a comforting and fragrant dessert.

Nutrition Information (per serving):

- Calories: 80
- Protein: 0g
- Carbohydrates: 22g

- Fat: 0g
- Fiber: 4g
- Sugar: 16g
- Portion size: 1 serving

Banana Nice Cream with Peanut Butter

Ingredients:

- 2 ripe bananas, sliced and frozen
- 2 tablespoons natural peanut butter
- Optional toppings: chopped nuts, cacao nibs, sliced banana

Instructions:

1. Place the frozen banana slices in a food processor or blender.
2. Add the peanut butter to the bananas.
3. Blend until smooth and creamy, scraping down the sides as needed.
4. Serve immediately as soft-serve ice cream or transfer to a container and freeze for a firmer texture.

5. Top with chopped nuts, cacao nibs, or sliced banana for extra flavor and crunch.

Nutrition Information (per serving):

- Calories: 220
- Protein: 5g
- Carbohydrates: 30g
- Fat: 10g
- Fiber: 4g
- Sugar: 16g
- Portion size: 1 serving

Coconut Flour Blueberry Muffins

Ingredients:

- 1/2 cup coconut flour
- 1/4 cup almond flour
- 1/4 teaspoon baking soda
- 1/4 teaspoon salt
- 3 eggs
- 1/4 cup coconut oil, melted
- 1/4 cup unsweetened almond milk
- 1/4 cup honey or maple syrup

- 1 teaspoon vanilla extract
- 1/2 cup fresh blueberries

Instructions:

1. Preheat the oven to 350°F (175°C) and line a muffin tin with paper liners.
2. In a large bowl, whisk together the coconut flour, almond flour, baking soda, and salt.
3. In a separate bowl, beat the eggs, then add the melted coconut oil, almond milk, honey or maple syrup, and vanilla extract. Mix well.
4. Pour the wet ingredients into the dry ingredients and stir until just combined.
5. Gently fold in the blueberries.
6. Divide the batter evenly among the muffin cups.
7. Bake for 20-25 minutes or until a toothpick inserted into the center comes out clean.
8. Allow the muffins to cool in the tin for 5 minutes before transferring to a wire rack to cool completely.

Nutrition Information (per muffin, makes 6 muffins):

- Calories: 200

- Protein: 5g

- Carbohydrates: 18g

- Fat: 13g

- Fiber: 4g

- Sugar: 12g

- Portion size: 1 muffin

Avocado Chocolate Mousse

Ingredients:

- 2 ripe avocados

- 1/4 cup unsweetened cocoa powder

- 1/4 cup honey or maple syrup

- 1 teaspoon vanilla extract

- Pinch of salt

- Optional toppings: sliced strawberries, whipped cream, chopped nuts

Instructions:

1. Scoop the flesh of the avocados into a food processor or blender.

2. Add the cocoa powder, honey or maple syrup, vanilla extract, and salt.

3. Blend until smooth and creamy, scraping down the sides as needed.

4. Transfer the mousse to serving dishes and refrigerate for at least 30 minutes to chill.

5. Serve topped with sliced strawberries, whipped cream, or chopped nuts for added indulgence.

Nutrition Information (per serving, makes 2 servings):

- Calories: 300
- Protein: 4g
- Carbohydrates: 28g
- Fat: 21g
- Fiber: 10g
- Sugar: 16g
- Portion size: 1 serving

Lemon Poppy Seed Cake Bites

Ingredients:

- 1 cup almond flour
- 1/4 cup coconut flour
- 1/4 cup powdered erythritol or stevia blend
- 2 tablespoons poppy seeds

- Zest of 1 lemon
- Juice of 1/2 lemon
- 1/4 cup coconut oil, melted
- 2 eggs
- 1 teaspoon vanilla extract
- 1/2 teaspoon baking soda
- Pinch of salt

Instructions:

1. Preheat the oven to 350°F (175°C) and line a baking sheet with parchment paper.
2. In a large bowl, combine the almond flour, coconut flour, powdered erythritol or stevia blend, poppy seeds, lemon zest, baking soda, and salt.
3. In a separate bowl, whisk together the melted coconut oil, eggs, lemon juice, and vanilla extract.
4. Pour the wet ingredients into the dry ingredients and mix until well combined.
5. Roll the dough into small balls and place them on the prepared baking sheet.
6. Flatten each ball slightly with the palm of your hand.

7. Bake for 10-12 minutes or until the edges are golden brown.

8. Allow the cake bites to cool on the baking sheet before serving.

Nutrition Information (per serving, makes 12 bites):

- Calories: 110

- Protein: 3g

- Carbohydrates: 6g

- Fat: 9g

- Fiber: 2g

- Sugar: 1g

- Portion size: 2 bites

Pistachlo Cranberry Energy Bites

Ingredients:

- 1 cup rolled oats

- 1/2 cup shelled pistachios, chopped

- 1/2 cup dried cranberries, chopped

- 1/4 cup almond butter

- 1/4 cup honey or maple syrup

- 1 teaspoon vanilla extract

- Pinch of salt

Instructions:

1. In a large bowl, combine the rolled oats, chopped pistachios, and dried cranberries.
2. In a small saucepan, heat the almond butter, honey or maple syrup, vanilla extract, and salt over low heat until smooth and well combined.
3. Pour the almond butter mixture over the dry ingredients and mix until evenly coated.
4. Roll the mixture into small balls and place them on a parchment-lined baking sheet.
5. Chill the energy bites in the refrigerator for at least 30 minutes before serving.

Nutrition Information (per serving, makes 12 bites):

- Calories: 130
- Protein: 3g
- Carbohydrates: 18g
- Fat: 6g
- Fiber: 2g
- Sugar: 9g

- Portion size: 2 bites

Pumpkin Pie Chia Pudding

Ingredients:

- 1/4 cup chia seeds
- 1 cup unsweetened almond milk
- 1/4 cup pumpkin puree
- 2 tablespoons maple syrup
- 1/2 teaspoon pumpkin pie spice
- 1/2 teaspoon vanilla extract

Instructions:

1. In a bowl, whisk together the chia seeds, almond milk, pumpkin puree, maple syrup, pumpkin pie spice, and vanilla extract.
2. Let the mixture sit for 5 minutes, then whisk again to prevent clumping.
3. Cover the bowl and refrigerate for at least 2 hours or overnight, until the pudding has thickened.
4. Serve the pumpkin pie chia pudding topped with a sprinkle of pumpkin pie spice for a festive touch.

Nutrition Information (per serving):

- Calories: 120
- Protein: 3g
- Carbohydrates: 15g
- Fat: 6g
- Fiber: 6g
- Sugar: 6g
- Portion size: 1 serving

Carrot Cake Oatmeal Cookies

Ingredients:

- 1 cup rolled oats
- 1/2 cup almond flour
- 1/4 cup shredded carrots
- 1/4 cup chopped walnuts
- 1/4 cup raisins
- 1/4 cup coconut oil, melted
- 1/4 cup honey or maple syrup
- 1 egg
- 1 teaspoon vanilla extract
- 1/2 teaspoon cinnamon
- Pinch of salt

Instructions:

1. Preheat the oven to 350°F (175°C) and line a baking sheet with parchment paper.
2. In a large bowl, combine the rolled oats, almond flour, shredded carrots, chopped walnuts, and raisins.
3. In a separate bowl, whisk together the melted coconut oil, honey or maple syrup, egg, vanilla extract, cinnamon, and salt.
4. Pour the wet ingredients into the dry ingredients and mix until well combined.
5. Drop spoonfuls of the cookie dough onto the prepared baking sheet.
6. Flatten each cookie slightly with the back of a spoon.
7. Bake for 10-12 minutes or until the edges are golden brown.
8. Allow the cookies to cool on the baking sheet for 5 minutes before transferring to a wire rack to cool completely.

Nutrition Information (per cookie, makes 12 cookies):

- Calories: 130
- Protein: 3g

- Carbohydrates: 15g

- Fat: 7g

- Fiber: 2g

- Sugar: 7g

- Portion size: 1 cookie

Chocolate Avocado Pudding

Ingredients:

- 2 ripe avocados

- 1/4 cup unsweetened cocoa powder

- 1/4 cup honey or maple syrup

- 1/4 cup unsweetened almond milk

- 1 teaspoon vanilla extract

- Pinch of salt

Instructions:

1. Scoop the flesh of the avocados into a food processor or blender.

2. Add the cocoa powder, honey or maple syrup, almond milk, vanilla extract, and salt.

3. Blend until smooth and creamy, scraping down the sides as needed.

4. Transfer the pudding to serving dishes and refrigerate for at least 30 minutes to chill.

5. Serve topped with shaved dark chocolate or sliced almonds for added texture.

Nutrition Information (per serving, makes 2 servings):

- Calories: 220
- Protein: 3g
- Carbohydrates: 25g
- Fat: 15g
- Fiber: 7g
- Sugar: 15g
- Portion size: 1 serving

These vibrant concoctions are not only delicious but also packed with essential nutrients to fuel your day. Whether you're looking for a quick breakfast option, a post-workout refuel, or a satisfying snack, these smoothie recipes have got you covered.

Green Smoothie with Spinach and Banana

Ingredients:

- 1 ripe banana
- 1 cup fresh spinach leaves
- 1/2 cup almond milk
- 1/2 cup Greek yogurt
- 1 tablespoon honey (optional)
- Ice cubes (optional)

Instructions:

1. Place all ingredients in a blender.
2. Blend until smooth and creamy.

3. Pour into a glass and enjoy!

Nutrition Information:

- Calories: 180
- Protein: 8g
- Carbohydrates: 30g
- Fat: 4g
- Fiber: 4g
- Sugar: 18g
- Portion size: 1 serving

Berry Blast Smoothie with Greek Yogurt

Ingredients:

- 1/2 cup mixed berries (strawberries, blueberries, raspberries)
- 1/2 cup Greek yogurt
- 1/2 cup almond milk
- 1 tablespoon honey (optional)
- Ice cubes (optional)

Instructions:

1. Combine all ingredients in a blender.
2. Blend until smooth and creamy.
3. Pour into a glass and enjoy!

Nutrition Information:

- Calories: 150
- Protein: 10g
- Carbohydrates: 25g
- Fat: 3g
- Fiber: 5g
- Sugar: 18g
- Portion size: 1 serving

Tropical Mango Pineapple Smoothie

Ingredients:

- 1/2 cup mango chunks
- 1/2 cup pineapple chunks
- 1/2 banana
- 1/2 cup coconut water
- Ice cubes (optional)

Instructions:

1. Add all ingredients to a blender.
2. Blend until smooth and creamy.
3. Serve immediately and enjoy!

Nutrition Information:

- Calories: 160
- Protein: 2g
- Carbohydrates: 40g
- Fat: 1g
- Fiber: 5g
- Sugar: 30g
- Portion size: 1 serving

Peanut Butter Banana Protein Smoothie

Ingredients:

- 1 ripe banana
- 2 tablespoons peanut butter
- 1 scoop protein powder (vanilla or chocolate)
- 1 cup almond milk

- Ice cubes (optional)

Instructions:

1. Combine all ingredients in a blender.
2. Blend until smooth and creamy.
3. Pour into a glass and enjoy!

Nutrition Information:

- Calories: 320
- Protein: 25g
- Carbohydrates: 25g
- Fat: 15g
- Fiber: 5g
- Sugar: 10g
- Portion size: 1 serving

Kale and Apple Detox Smoothie

Ingredients:

- 1 cup kale leaves, stems removed
- 1 green apple, cored and chopped
- 1/2 cucumber, chopped
- Juice of 1/2 lemon

- 1/2 cup coconut water

- Ice cubes (optional)

Instructions:

1. Place all ingredients in a blender.

2. Blend until smooth and well combined.

3. Pour into a glass and enjoy!

Nutrition Information:

- Calories: 120

- Protein: 3g

- Carbohydrates: 25g

- Fat: 1g

- Fiber: 7g

- Sugar: 15g

- Portion size: 1 serving

Blueberry Avocado Smoothie

Ingredients:

- 1/2 cup blueberries

- 1/2 ripe avocado

- 1/2 cup spinach leaves

- 1/2 cup Greek yogurt
- 1/2 cup almond milk
- Ice cubes (optional)

Instructions:

1. Combine all ingredients in a blender.
2. Blend until smooth and creamy.
3. Pour into a glass and enjoy!

Nutrition Information:

- Calories: 220
- Protein: 10g
- Carbohydrates: 25g
- Fat: 10g
- Fiber: 8g
- Sugar: 15g
- Portion size: 1 serving

Chocolate Banana Protein Smoothie

Ingredients:

- 1 ripe banana
- 1 tablespoon cocoa powder

- 1 scoop chocolate protein powder
- 1 cup unsweetened almond milk
- Ice cubes (optional)

Instructions:

1. Place all ingredients in a blender.
2. Blend until smooth and creamy.
3. Serve immediately and enjoy!

Nutrition Information:

- Calories: 280
- Protein: 20g
- Carbohydrates: 30g
- Fat: 8g
- Fiber: 6g
- Sugar: 12g
- Portion size: 1 serving

Beet and Berry Smoothie

Ingredients:

- 1/2 cup cooked beets, chopped

- 1/2 cup mixed berries (strawberries, raspberries, blueberries)
- 1/2 cup Greek yogurt
- 1/2 cup almond milk
- Ice cubes (optional)

Instructions:

1. Combine all ingredients in a blender.
2. Blend until smooth and well combined.
3. Pour into a glass and enjoy!

Nutrition Information:

- Calories: 150
- Protein: 8g
- Carbohydrates: 25g
- Fat: 2g
- Fiber: 6g
- Sugar: 15g
- Portion size: 1 serving

Peach and Almond Smoothie

Ingredients:

- 1 ripe peach, pitted and chopped
- 1/4 cup almonds
- 1/2 cup Greek yogurt
- 1/2 cup almond milk
- Ice cubes (optional)

Instructions:

1. Add all ingredients to a blender.
2. Blend until smooth and creamy.
3. Serve immediately and enjoy!

Nutrition Information:

- Calories: 240
- Protein: 12g
- Carbohydrates: 30g
- Fat: 10g
- Fiber: 5g
- Sugar: 20g
- Portion size: 1 serving

Spinach and Pineapple Smoothie

Ingredients:

- 1 cup fresh spinach leaves
- 1/2 cup pineapple chunks
- 1/2 banana
- 1/2 cup coconut water
- Ice cubes (optional)

Instructions:

1. Place all ingredients in a blender.
2. Blend until smooth and creamy.
3. Pour into a glass and enjoy!

Nutrition Information:

- Calories: 140
- Protein: 3g
- Carbohydrates: 30g
- Fat: 1g
- Fiber: 5g
- Sugar: 20g
- Portion size: 1 serving

Coconut Watermelon Smoothie

Ingredients:

- 1 cup watermelon cubes
- 1/2 cup coconut water
- Juice of 1 lime
- 1 tablespoon honey (optional)
- Ice cubes (optional)

Instructions:

1. Combine all ingredients in a blender.
2. Blend until smooth and well combined.
3. Serve immediately and enjoy!

Nutrition Information:

- Calories: 90
- Protein: 1g
- Carbohydrates: 25g
- Fat: 0g
- Fiber: 1g
- Sugar: 20g
- Portion size: 1 serving

Carrot Cake Smoothie

Ingredients:

- 1/2 cup shredded carrots
- 1/2 banana
- 1/4 cup rolled oats
- 1/2 teaspoon cinnamon
- 1 cup almond milk
- Ice cubes (optional)

Instructions:

1. Add all ingredients to a blender.
2. Blend until smooth and creamy.
3. Pour into a glass and enjoy!

Nutrition Information:

- Calories: 180
- Protein: 5g
- Carbohydrates: 35g
- Fat: 3g
- Fiber: 5g
- Sugar: 15g
- Portion size: 1 serving

Mango Coconut Smoothie Bowl

Ingredients:

- 1 ripe mango, peeled and chopped
- 1/2 cup coconut milk
- 1/4 cup Greek yogurt
- 1/4 cup shredded coconut
- Ice cubes (optional)
- Toppings: sliced banana, granola, chia seeds

Instructions:

1. Combine mango, coconut milk, Greek yogurt, and shredded coconut in a blender.
2. Blend until smooth and creamy.
3. Pour the smoothie into a bowl.
4. Add your favorite toppings such as sliced banana, granola, and chia seeds.
5. Serve immediately and enjoy!

Nutrition Information:

- Calories: 280
- Protein: 5g
- Carbohydrates: 30g

- Fat: 18g

- Fiber: 6g

- Sugar: 25g

- Portion size: 1 serving

Cucumber Mint Smoothie

Ingredients:

- 1/2 cucumber, peeled and chopped

- Handful of fresh mint leaves

- Juice of 1 lime

- 1 cup coconut water

- Ice cubes (optional)

Instructions:

1. Place cucumber, mint leaves, lime juice, and coconut water in a blender.

2. Blend until smooth.

3. Add ice cubes if desired and blend again until well combined.

4. Pour into a glass and serve immediately.

Nutrition Information:

- Calories: 70
- Protein: 2g
- Carbohydrates: 15g
- Fat: 0g
- Fiber: 3g
- Sugar: 8g
- Portion size: 1 serving

Orange Creamsicle Smoothie

Ingredients:

- 1 large orange, peeled and segmented
- 1/2 cup Greek yogurt
- 1/2 cup almond milk
- 1 tablespoon honey (optional)
- Ice cubes (optional)

Instructions:

1. Combine orange segments, Greek yogurt, almond milk, and honey in a blender.
2. Blend until smooth and creamy.

3. Add ice cubes if desired and blend again until well combined.

4. Pour into a glass and enjoy!

Nutrition Information:

- Calories: 150

- Protein: 8g

- Carbohydrates: 25g

- Fat: 2g

- Fiber: 4g

- Sugar: 18g

- Portion size: 1 serving

CONCLUSION

"The Type 1 Diabetes Cookbook for Adults" serves as a culinary compass, guiding individuals with type 1 diabetes on a journey towards flavorful, nutritious, and blood sugar-friendly meals. Throughout these pages, we've delved into the intricate dance between food and insulin, offering not just recipes, but a comprehensive approach to managing diabetes through mindful eating.

As we bid adieu, remember that this book is not just a collection of recipes; it's a testament to the power of choice and control over one's health. Each dish is crafted with care, balancing taste with nutritional integrity, empowering you to savor the richness of life without compromising on well-being.

But our journey together doesn't end here. It's merely the beginning of a lifelong culinary adventure, where you'll continue to explore, experiment, and evolve in your quest for optimal health. Armed with knowledge, creativity, and the unwavering spirit of resilience, you're equipped to navigate the complexities of diabetes with grace and determination.

So here's to you, the intrepid chef of your own destiny. May your kitchen be a sanctuary of healing, your table a celebration of vitality, and your heart a beacon of hope for a brighter, healthier tomorrow. Cheers to good food, good health, and the boundless possibilities that lie ahead.

www.ingramcontent.com/pod-product-compliance
Lightning Source LLC
Chambersburg PA
CBHW071008250726
48653CB00005B/1559